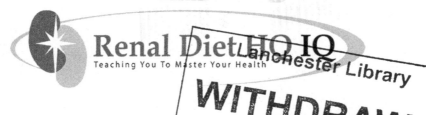

Renal Diet HQ IQ
Teaching You To Master Your Health

The Emotional Challenges Of Coping with Chronic Kidney Disease

By Mathea Ford, RD/LD

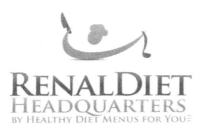

RENALDIET
HEADQUARTERS
BY HEALTHY DIET MENUS FOR YOU

Page | 2

Purpose and Introduction

What I have found through the emails and requests of my readers is that it is difficult to find information about a pre-dialysis kidney diet that is actionable. I want you to know that is what I intend to provide in all my books.

I wrote this book with you in mind: the person with kidney problems who does not know where to start or can't seem to get the answers that you need from other sources. This book will provide information that is applicable to a predialysis kidney disease diet.

Who am I? I am a registered dietitian in the USA who has been working with kidney patients for my entire 15 + years of experience. Find all my books on Amazon on my author page: http://www.amazon.com/Mathea-Ford/e/B008E1E7IS/

My goals are simple – to give some answers and to create an understanding of what is typical. In this series of 12 books, I will take you through the different parts of being a person with pre-dialysis kidney disease. It will not necessarily be what happens in your case, as everyone is an individual. I may simplify things in an effort to write them so that I feel you can learn the most from the information. This may mean that I don't say the exact things that your doctor would say. If you don't understand, please ask your doctor.

I want you to know, I am not a medical doctor and I am not aware of your particular condition. Information in this book is current as of publication, but may or may not have changed. This book is not meant to substitute for medical treatment for you, your friends, your caregivers, or your family members. You should not base treatment decisions solely on what is contained in this book. Develop your treatment plan with your doctors, nurses and the other medical professionals on your team. I recommend that you double-check any information with your medical team to verify if it applies to you.

In other words, I am not responsible for your medical care. I am providing this book for information and entertainment purposes, not medical diagnoses. Please consult with your doctor about any questions that you have about your particular case.

Table of Contents

Coping With A Chronic Illness

Nearly half of all people living in the United States live with a chronic illness. A chronic illness is defined as a medical condition that can be controlled, but not cured. Chronic kidney disease is one such chronic illness and affects a large portion of the population. According to the Centers for Disease Control and Prevention, 1 in 10 American adults have some level of chronic kidney disease. That adds up to more than 20 million people in the United States alone.

Living with a chronic condition such as chronic kidney disease has both physical and emotional ramifications for the individual, as well as for the people around them. The physical symptoms are often quiet until you reach the later stages of the disease. The emotional symptoms, however, are vast and can be seen very early on. It's an emotional journey that can include changing relationships, complicated decisions, and uncertainty of the future. It is also a progressive disease that can affect your caregivers as well as yourself.

There are three forms of kidney disease: hereditary, congenital, and acquired. Hereditary kidney disease is something that was inherited through the genes. One of the most frequently found forms of inherited kidney disease is Polycystic Kidney Disease (PKD). With congenital kidney disease there were malformations in the kidney and possibly other surrounding organs that were present at birth. The most common kind of kidney disease is acquired. Acquired kidney disease was not present at birth and is usually chronic. It is not always known why a person develops kidney disease.

Like other chronic illnesses, chronic kidney disease can be progressive. Because the condition is usually irreversible, it's generally something that must be lived with and dealt with for life. In the late stages of chronic kidney disease, end-stage renal disease (ESRD) can occur and that requires dialysis or even a kidney transplant. Many patients opt for a transplant, but even that is not an entirely permanent option since it entails more medications and heightened health awareness. You may require dialysis while you are waiting on a transplant.

Due to the fact that symptoms of chronic kidney disease are not always present and visible it's considered an "invisible illness". Most people can't tell you have it just by looking at you, but psychological and emotional impact of discovering your diagnosis can be devastating. In addition, most individuals with chronic kidney disease find that they must make changes to their lifestyle.

Chronic kidney disease can affect almost every aspect of a person's body and lead to everything from damage to the nervous system to impotence and anemia. It can even cause degenerative bone disease and an impaired immune system. Dealing with all of these setbacks and challenges can be difficult and overwhelming, even for someone who normally has a fairly healthy and positive outlook on life. Symptoms can include fatigue, weakness, loss of appetite, and insomnia. Any one of these can have an effect on your psychological health and lead to additional symptoms and effects for which you might not have been ready.

Even with a diagnosis of chronic kidney disease, it is still possible to lead a fulfilling and rewarding life. By practicing good self-care and working with your doctors to find the best treatment and care it's even possible to experience an overall good quality of life. In the following chapters we will discuss how living with a chronic illness can affect your life, or a loved one's, and some measures you can take to overcome the various challenges that present themselves. Although it's not always an easy ride and there are many obstacles that often need to be overcome, you can still enjoy your life and beat the odds by gaining little victories and engaging in a positive approach to your happiness.

The Initial Shock

Every day millions of people are challenged to cope with a debilitating chronic illness. In many cases, the treatment options can be as challenging as the illness itself. Along with the physical manifestations of the illness, there are also changes that can be social too. Living with a chronic illness such as kidney disease presents challenges that "healthy" people just can't begin to understand.

In addition to suffering from the physical impacts of kidney disease, other areas of life such as jobs, recreational pursuits, and social activities can be affected. Emotional tolls don't only fall on the individual suffering from kidney disease but can also impact family, friends, and the people around them.

Many people, upon hearing the diagnosis of their chronic illness, may begin experiencing depression, anxiety, and other emotions that can be difficult to deal with. As the person being diagnosed with chronic kidney disease, you might also go through the five stages of grief as you grieve the "old you" and start learning how to live with your "new normal." It's natural to grieve for the healthy individual that you'll never completely be again. It's also possible that you will continue to learn new ways to cope with the ongoing effects of chronic kidney disease. This might require constant reorganizing and redefinition of yourself based on the new reality that the illness imposes.

Getting the initial diagnosis can be quite a shock, especially if you are without any symptoms. Some people find that they feel powerless and that the disease itself almost takes on a life of its own. It's easy to feel out of control of your own body at a time like this. It's important, however, to learn that you do still have control over most areas of your life and that you are still able to make decisions that can affect your quality of life.

Due to the complex nature of the disease, it can be overwhelming to have a lot of information come your way. Many people are diagnosed with chronic kidney disease and had very little knowledge about it prior to their diagnosis. Learning about the treatment options available, the related medical conditions, and the details about the disease can be a daunting task.

Getting The News

Without a doubt, getting the news of your diagnosis can be one of the most unsettling experiences that you will ever encounter.

In the early stages of chronic kidney disease, most people are actually unaware their kidneys are even damaged. Because they have millions of nephrons, which are the tiny structures inside the kidneys that filter your blood, having just a few damaged ones normally won't have much effect on the kidneys' capacity to function. However, because chronic kidney disease is progressive, over time more nephrons can become damaged until the last ones may be unable to efficiently filter the wastes and excess fluid from the bloodstream. Since this happens over time, you may find that it may take as long as 20 years before it progresses to end stage renal disease.

In the beginning, it's normal to feel a certain amount of shock and disbelief. Although some people do panic, others feel like they're watching the scene with detachment, as though they are viewing a television show or someone else's life. The shock might just last a few minutes or as long as several weeks. Of course, it's not possible to deny that you do have a serious medical condition, especially if you do have symptoms. Especially in the later stages of kidney disease, it's important that you act quickly on any available treatment options in order to sustain your kidney function.

Some people, upon learning that they have chronic kidney disease, push against the diagnosis and continue challenging their body in ways that they did in the past-or maybe even *more* so. This is an attempt to prove to themselves that they are "okay" and that there really isn't anything seriously wrong. This resistance is not uncommon. Unfortunately, it can also cause exhaustion which can lead to a sudden decline in your condition, often called crashing.

Feelings of fear and anxiety are common upon getting the news of your diagnosis. The future seems uncertain and you might experience feelings of hopelessness and grief. In fact, many people go through the five stages of grief as they learn to adjust to the news and their new way of living.

Stages Of Grief

In 1969, Elizabeth Kubler-Ross developed the five stages of grief to explain the different stages that someone who has lost a loved one might face, but it also applies to someone who has been diagnosed with a chronic illness. Since their introduction, the stages have evolved. Although there is no typical case, since all individuals are different, the model does offer some insight into the grieving process.

The five stages are comprised of: denial, anger, bargaining, depression, and acceptance. Not everyone goes through all of them and the stages themselves are not necessarily gone through in order. You might, for instance, go through depression for a long time and then find yourself angry again before moving into acceptance. It is even possible to enter the acceptance stage and stay there, only to find yourself feeling depressed as over time your illness progresses.

Denial

Denial is normally the first stage that you go through after you learn about your diagnosis. Shock can also be included in this stage. Denial is really your body's way of trying to help you grasp the message and deal with the shock of the news that you received. When things get too overwhelming and you can't make sense of what is going on, the mind tends to try to ignore the stressors and this is where denial comes into play. Some people also describe it as "going numb".

If you go through denial, you might find yourself using avoidance strategies. Those who use these kinds of tactics tend to ask very few questions about their medical condition. They aren't interested in hearing about the treatment options or what might happen to them on down the road. They might tune the doctor out while he is talking or brush the news off as though it isn't that important. They aren't motivated to try to make any lifestyle changes, such as following a different diet, and they don't want to hear about long-term treatment options that sound scary, like dialysis and surgery.

Once you start accepting the reality of your diagnosis, begin asking questions, and seeking answers, you're actually starting the healing part of the grief process. When you leave the denial stage you do become stronger and take on more coping mechanisms. Sometimes the feelings that you were trying to ignore will begin to surface and become more visible.

Anger

Anger is one of the most prominent stages of the grieving process and the stage that most people will be able to relate to at one time or another. It might be the stage that others around you find the most difficult to deal with, but it is a necessary stage of the healing process. It's important to feel your anger and not ignore it. The more you acknowledge your anger and deal with it the more quickly it will start to go away.

Anger comes up in the grieving process because it's an emotion that is familiar and easier to process. Many people feel angry before they feel anything else. Anger can be directed at many different things, or people, in your life but it's generally standing in front of another emotion. You might, for instance, feel hopeless or helpless but since your mind isn't ready to deal with those emotions yet, anger covers them up. After a diagnosis of chronic illness, many people feel alone. Their mind tells them to be angry at those around them for not being there (when in fact the other people in their life really are being supportive in the best ways they know how). Anger can also eventually offer structure to your feelings and make them more identifiable.

It's easy to look at your situation and ask *why me?* The fact that there may not be a solid reason for you to have chronic kidney disease can be frustrating. It feels very unfair. Anger can be destructive, both to your emotional health and to the people around you. If you express yourself in anger too often then you might alienate those who care about you, leaving you feeling even more isolated and alone.

On the other hand, anger does have some benefits. Anger can help you get your feelings out and open up communication. You can't control how you feel, but you can control how you deal with those feelings. Look for some ways to let your anger be productive if you can.

Bargaining

Bargaining, like denial, is the mind's attempt at controlling and minimizing the situation. When we are given bad news, part of our mind doesn't want to believe it. It needs more time to process the information. Your mind doesn't really believe in the severity of your situation. Instead of coping with the news in a realistic way, it believes that the situation can be fixed.

You might find that once you have been diagnosed with chronic kidney disease you try to bargain your way out of the severity of the illness. Rather than facing what you're really going through you might, for instance, appeal to your own body (or doctor) and promise to take better care of your health, eat more vegetables, and get more exercise if the illness will just go away.

Likewise, part of bargaining includes hindsight guilt. Instead of thinking about the future and how you might change your habits in order to avoid the severity of your chronic illness you might think about the past and start regretting the choices you made that might have led to this diagnosis. Guilt is regularly found alongside of bargaining. Thinking about the "what ifs" can cause you to find fault in yourself and what you believe you could have done differently. You might attempt to negotiate with your doctors, with your body, or even with your past self in an effort to try and avoid the reality of your situation.

Depression

Once you do begin to accept the reality of your situation and what the future might hold for you, you might face depression. Depression usually lasts longer than the previous stages and can return again even after you've moved on into acceptance. The grief that is depression is actually a completely normal and even appropriate response to a great loss. It is important to remember that receiving a diagnosis of chronic kidney disease really does constitute as a great loss since it means that your life will no longer be what it once was. (That doesn't mean that you can't have a fulfilling life!)

In depression you might find yourself withdrawing from family and friends, ignoring social occasions, and living in a fog of powerful sadness. You might wonder if it's even worth continuing on with your life. Although the depression stage can be scary, it's natural and an important part of the healing process since it allows you to grieve for the things that you might no longer be able to do and express sadness at the fact that your life is changing.

It's important to understand that sadness is different from depression. Most people assume that you're going to be sad from time to time as you are dealing with your illness. However, sadness can be fleeting and irregular. Sadness can help bring tears and allow you to emotionally cope with how you are feeling. Once the moment has passed, or you've talked to someone else, the sadness usually goes away. However, with depression you never really feel yourself feeling better. You might feel helpless, hopeless, and isolated but in depression these feelings might not ever go away. It can interfere with your daily activities and affect your relationships, and you may need to ask for help from your healthcare team to deal with this.

Acceptance

Some people mistakenly confuse acceptance with being "okay". Acceptance does not mean that you are okay with your illness and that everything is going to be alright. In fact, you'll probably never feel *good* about having a chronic illness and most people would rather have the news reversed and never have to deal with being sick at all.

What acceptance really means is that you understand that what you are dealing with now is a permanent reality. Although you might not like the new reality that you are living in, you understand that you're going to have to accept your limitations and be joyful for what you have. Choices need to be made as your health condition changes. You might re-learn new organizational skills, reorganize roles, and even learn how to express yourself in a different way. In acceptance, you can learn to forge new meaningful relationships, enjoy a different kind of quality of life, and even evolve with new understanding and insight.

As your health condition changes you might revisit the other stages of grief. As chronic kidney disease can be progressive, you might find that you are experiencing more symptoms and need to make more changes to your lifestyle. When this happens, you might go back to feeling angry or depressed all over again as your mind tries to acclimate itself to your body's changes.

Telling Others

After you find out the news regarding your diagnosis it's then up to you to tell the other people in your life about what is going on. Telling those who are closest to you can be extremely difficult and dealing with the consequences of the possible changes in the relationship dynamics afterwards can be even more challenging.

Your partner

As the person who probably knows you the most intimately, telling your partner about your chronic illness might be one of the most complicated tasks you face. If he/she accompanies you to your doctor's appointment, then breaking the news will come to both of you at the same time. If you're left to tell your partner on your own, however, finding the words to let them know that you are suffering from chronic kidney disease may not come easy.

Sharing the news is difficult on more than one level. Not only will the news be unsettling because they care about you; it might also become the moment when you both realize that he/she might one day have to become your caregiver. Not only is your life potentially going to change, but *his/her* life might also be headed in another direction as well.

You shouldn't be surprised if your partner reacts to your news in the same way in which you did. They might express shock, disbelief, and sadness. They might also express anger and resentment, even though it isn't directed at you.

Some people find that their partner shows avoidance and doesn't want to hear the specifics involved in the information pertaining to kidney disease. They might not want to hear about the treatment options and the severity of your condition because they might feel like the knowledge makes your condition too much of a reality.

Your co-workers

Depending on the type of kidney disease you have, you may find that you must miss work for doctor appointments and tests. You might also suffer from fatigue and other symptoms that can make it more difficult to perform your duties as you once did. As your illness progresses you might not be able to perform the same job functions as you once did. You might not be able to work at all.

What you tell your co-workers and when you tell them is up to you. You might tell one co-worker with whom you are close and leave the general announcement until the progression reaches a level where it's unavoidable to let others around you know. A lot of people feel if they are able to perform their job duties, they don't need to tell their co-workers about their medical conditions. They don't want to receive special treatment or risk being terminated.

On the other hand, you might also tell your co-workers about your diagnosis and find that you are able to receive a lot of support from the people with whom you spend most of your day. Your own individual working situation will really dictate whom you tell and how much you disclose.

If you disclose your illness and your supervisor questions your job performance, then you can assure them that you don't expect any problems. You can always revisit this issue at another time, if a problem does arise. Of course, if you do need to make some adjustments then it's best to upfront and honest. You might find that your workplace is more than happy to accommodate you when possible.

Your parents

As a child it was your parents who probably made you feel better when you were under the weather. Your parents loved you and protected you. Just because you're an adult does not mean that the protectiveness has left them. Even though they understand that you are a responsible and capable adult, it doesn't mean that they don't still have the urge to shield you and try to make everything better.

With that in mind, when a parent learns that their child has a chronic illness the news can be devastating. Not being able to "fix" you and protect you from the effects of your illness can be depressing and overwhelming.

Some people find when they tell their parents about their diagnosis, the immediate reaction is to question the doctor's credentials, ask for a second opinion, and/or criticize any test results or analysis that was done. This, in its own way, is a form of denial since the disbelief is so present. Even though you are an adult, parents still want the best for you and learning that you have a medical condition that they have no control over can be devastating.

Your children

If you have older children who communicate well, and you have to attend regular treatments (like dialysis) and doctors' appointments, you might wish to discuss your diagnosis with them. They will almost certainly want to know if you are going to be okay and if your life is in danger. They might also ask if there is a chance that they will become sick, too, and wonder how their lives will be impacted by your diagnosis. If you have younger children, you might need to simplify your language and stick to the facts. Older children might be capable of understanding more, so take your children's age into consideration.

It's important for your children to be able to ask questions and for you to help them understand the answers. Children seek stability and the idea of their lives being overturned by something is scary, even to the older and more independent child. You, as their parent, are part of their foundation and when this is threatened children can become scared and feel defenseless.

When you first tell your children about your illness, be prepared to be met with lots of questions. On the flip side, your child might not react at all. They might change the subject and act as if nothing is wrong. This doesn't mean they don't care. This may be their way of showing denial. They might just be trying to process the news and could return to you later for another conversation about it.

Your friends

When you inform your friends of your diagnosis, you can be sure to get varied and even unpredictable reactions. Some will react flatly and almost act as though the news you're sharing isn't as big of a deal as it actually is. Others might react more excitedly, shocked and dismayed at what you are telling them. You'll also have a few middle-of-the-road reactions.

It's important not to assume that an unemotional response from a friend means that they aren't taking your chronic kidney disease diagnosis seriously. Some people simply need time to process the news and think about it before they are able to absorb the information. Imagine a conversation that goes like this:

You: I've been diagnosed with chronic kidney disease.

Friend: Really? Oh, that's too bad. Listen, did you catch the last episode of...

A reaction (or non-reaction) like this can be hurtful. Try not to take it personally. In fact, you might discover that days or even weeks after you share the news with them, they contact you and sound more upset at your diagnosis than they initially did.

You might find that some friends take the news very hard. This can be challenging as well since it means you might have to comfort your friend; an ironic role since it feels like they should be the one to comfort you. Although this type of reaction might feel unfair, it also means that your friend needs time to adjust to the news and cares about you very much. If you find that you have to comfort them too much, and that it takes a lot of your time and emotional energy, then you might want to distance yourself until they've had time to process your news.

Almost everyone will have at least a few basic questions about your diagnosis. You should be prepared to meet their questions with at least a few basic facts about your pain, treatment options, and prognosis. You can also encourage them to learn more on their own and even point them in the direction of a few good websites should they desire to conduct their own research.

It is not necessary to share your diagnosis and your health status with everybody you know. Of course, you can if you want to. If you do not want everyone to know, however, then when you tell someone of your condition, make it clear to them that it's a delicate situation and you'd be pleased if details of your condition weren't publicly shared. Remember that every time you tell another person there is always that chance that the news and facts will be repeated to someone else. And the "facts" about your diagnosis may change as the information passes from person to person over time.

Admitting You're Sick

After you've had time to process the fact that you've been diagnosed and you've shared the news with those closest to you, it's time to address the situation of your emotional self. Admitting to yourself that you're actually sick and finding your "new normal" is not easy. In fact, telling *yourself* that you're sick is sometimes harder than telling anyone else.

Finding Your New Normal

With time your kidney disease will be part of you, and you will have a "new normal". What is a "new normal?" The new normal simply means the way that you carry on with your life. Living with kidney disease affects every part of your life and your significant relationships.

You might be shocked when you first learn that you have a chronic medical condition. One question that many people ask of themselves is "why me?" You might wonder where it came from and why you have the condition when others in similar shape as you don't have it. Unfortunately, there might not ever be a good answer to this question. Although there are conditions that can greatly increase the chance of developing chronic kidney disease, sometimes a person can be diagnosed with it and have nothing that would have indicated a predisposition.

You'll probably begin your journey by learning as much about chronic kidney disease as you can. Many people spend countless hours researching their disease, treatment options, and symptoms in order to become more familiar with what is happening to their body.

Although it's better to be informed, sometimes the more you know about your condition the more overwhelmed you might feel. You could begin the grieving process again. You might feel angry that you have the disease and/or sad because you understand that you might not be able to live in the same way that you were used to living. You might also feel overwhelmed and stressed at the idea of learning new ways to take care of yourself or at the thought of a loved one becoming burdened with you and your needs.

Discovering Limitations

One of the first things that you might fear upon getting a diagnosis of a chronic illness is that you may not be able to do the things you love or enjoy a high standard of living anymore. Although there are limitations that you might have with chronic kidney disease, it is possible to learn new ways of doing things so that these limitations are not confining.

It is important to learn how to live with chronic kidney disease. At first you might feel as though you are no longer a complete person and that your condition is controlling you. The more you learn to live with it, though, the more in control you'll feel and the more you'll be able to adjust to your new normal.

Sometimes, learning about your illness and gaining knowledge can help in this area. Although you'll certainly discover lots of limitations as you're doing research, keep in mind that not all of the limitations are going to apply to you and your situation. Also remember that not all internet information is reliable so if you come across something that sounds really frightening and overwhelming then be sure to check it against another source. Talk to your doctor if you have any questions.

Part of your new normal might mean that you have to stick to a healthier diet than you've had in the past. Adding renal diet specific items to your diet might be difficult if it's not something you are used to. You might also have dietary restrictions: sodium, potassium, phosphorus, and protein can be limited in a renal diet. Over time, however, this will become your new normal.

You might also have medications that you need to take on a daily basis. Although sticking to a medication schedule and remembering to take your medicine every day can feel overwhelming in the beginning, soon it will become routine.

5 Ways to Remember Your Medications

1. Make a chart and hang it on your refrigerator. Cross off the medications as you take them.

2. Take the same medications at the same time every day.

3. Place your medication next to something you use every day, like your computer. It will act as a visual reminder.

4. Set an alarm in your house that will remind you when it's time to take your medication.

5. Ask someone to help you remember, such as your spouse or a roommate.

Moving Into Acceptance

Finding your new normal is an important part of the grieving process since it helps you move into acceptance. Along the way, you truly have to be gentle with yourself. Understand that you will learn to adapt over time. The first year is always the hardest. Although you might not ever completely feel like your old self again, you can learn to fit your condition into your life and find a new way of living that is just as good-if not better.

The confusion that you might feel in the beginning as you are learning to adapt will eventually get better. As you learn to adjust yourself to your limitations and find different ways of approaching things that you did in the past you'll feel less overwhelmed. It is very important to take your time and learn how to take care of both your mental and physical needs.

Coping Emotionally With Kidney Disease

Oftentimes, coping with the physical problems of chronic kidney disease is easier than coping with the emotional issues. Most of the issues concerning chronic kidney disease are physical. However, any time you suffer from a chronic illness there are emotional concerns. It is imperative to address your emotional health and treat it as carefully as you do your physical health.

Physical Discomfort, Emotional Pain

It might be the physical discomfort from chronic kidney disease that you were prepared to face, but it could be the emotional pain that is tougher. With end stage renal failure, there are many symptoms that you might have to face. These can include: fatigue, disorientation, anxiety, tremors, itching, weight changes, and breathing changes. Some emotions aren't always easy to identify. For instance, you might find that you're irritable or that you want to sleep a lot. These can be signs of depression. It is also extremely common to feel stressed or overwhelmed as you attempt to coordinate your daily living with the new limitations and nuances that living with chronic kidney disease can bring.

The uncertainty of chronic kidney disease can have a significant impact on your emotional health. You might discover that you feel good for awhile and then your condition changes, leaving you feeling weakened and sick. This can cause you to feel out of control of your body and your life.

Daily living may become difficult. You might experience diminished performance at work and at home. Many people find that sticking to a renal diet can make eating out difficult. This can make some social situations uncomfortable. The fatigue that often comes with chronic kidney disease might make you feel exhausted all the time, thus limiting the amount of physical activity you do. You might also have to depend on someone to help see to your basic needs and this reliance can be embarrassing and stressful.

Keeping Positive

After the diagnosis of a chronic illness there can be new emotions and feelings that must be dealt with-some of which you may have never experienced. If you're the type of person who has always felt positive and well-adjusted then suddenly feeling stressed and anxious might be unsettling. Likewise, if you were always full of a lot of energy and active then dealing with the fatigue and physical pain of kidney disease can make you feel depressed.

Being gentle with yourself is one of the keys to staying positive. Part of being gentle with yourself means giving yourself permission to feel the feelings you are having. It's okay to feel bad and to feel negative from time to time. When you must deal with challenges on a daily basis it's hard to constantly stay positive. Giving into your sadness and anger and anxiety on a limited basis is normal and healthy. You might feel ashamed or even guilty about feeling angry, especially if you think others might have it worse off. Remember that you are human, and don't discount your feelings.

Coping with the mental and emotional challenges of chronic kidney disease requires a positive, yet realistic, approach. You *can* find a happy, fulfilling life with the diagnosis of chronic kidney disease. In fact, a recent study of kidney patients undergoing multiple dialysis treatments discovered that their perceived mood and life satisfaction wasn't any different from a control group of healthy people.

When you're living with a chronic medical condition, keeping an eternally optimistic outlook is almost impossible. Your disease is scary, especially if you are facing one of the later stages of it. It forces you to deal with uncertainty. You no longer have complete control over your life. But your doctors are there to help you.

For those facing a chronic condition, it's hard when the people in their lives continuously encourage them to feel positive or happy. When someone says something like, "Everything happens for a reason," or makes another cheery remark it can put pressure on you to act positive, even when you don't feel like it.

Instead of ignoring your hardships and feelings, acknowledge them. That is a big part in learning to love yourself with your illness. When you're struggling with something then acknowledging how hard your situation is can be the first step in learning to cope with it.

Gaining A Positive Outlook

Your outlook on life can reduce or increase the symptoms that can be associated with chronic kidney disease and other related conditions, including diabetes, heart disease, and high blood pressure. A recent study from the Weill Cornell Medical College discovered that how people relate to their pain can either help or hinder healthy coping. The report, published in the September 2010 issue of Psychology and Aging (Vol. 25, No. 3), found that a person's habitual outlook on life and their ability to sustain positive emotions in the face of adversity or stress can make a difference in their experience of chronic pain.

The report also found that those who have an exaggerated negative view of the actual or anticipated pain makes the experience of pain worse. It can contribute to increased pain severity, disability, and emotional distress and lead to anxiety and worry.

15 Ways to Keep a Positive Outlook

1. **Manage your stress**. Your emotional and mental state are important when you're dealing with a chronic illness. Emotional pain is related to physical pain and if you can deal with your stress in healthy ways then you can effectively deal with your other symptoms as well.

2. **It's just temporary**. Although your chronic illness isn't going to go away, unfortunately, the symptom that you're experiencing at the moment is usually temporary. You might feel fatigued right now, but you could have a good day tomorrow and feel energized. Few things are ever completely permanent. Having hope that even something big will somehow get better, or ease up, is a step in becoming more positive.

3. **Make connections**. Connecting with others who understand what you're going through and can sympathize with you is important. There is only so

much that family and friends can do and sometimes you need to find others who are coming from the same place as you are. Look for support online in health-related communities or talk to your doctor about local support groups.

4. **Control your attitude**. You might not have any control over your symptoms or the progress that your disease is making, but you have control over your attitude. You can choose to be positive. This doesn't mean that you can't still have bad days and moments, but when you're thinking long-term, think positive.

5. **Look beyond your illness**. By continuing to enjoy life outside of your illness you are proving that you are more than just chronic kidney disease. You are still YOU! This might mean finding new hobbies, making new connections, or reorganizing your normal activities to make them more comfortable but make sure you're still living to the best of your abilities.

6. **See to your needs**. Make sure you take care of yourself and are getting enough to eat on your renal diet, drink, and sleep. Don't underestimate the effects that lack of sleep and a poor diet can have on your mental and physical health.

7. **See other people**. Try to stay connected to friends and family members. Healthy, positive interpersonal relationships can be good for your mental health.

8. **Have a routine.** A routine offers stability which can bring a sense of control and order in your life.

9. **Feel good about your doctor**. In fact, make sure you have a doctor you trust. Good rapport is just as important as having a knowledgeable doctor. Your relationship with your doctor is critical to your health.

10. **Be honest**. When it comes to your feelings and how you are doing, be honest with yourself and those close to you. Holding it inside can make things worse.

11. **Be gentle with yourself**. Sometimes it helps to create a new measuring stick. If you compare your "new normal" to your old self, it can be depressing. Instead, find new ways of measuring your success and quality of life. For instance, instead of feeling good about yourself after running 5 miles, recalculate your expectations and feel good about yourself when you only run 2 miles.

12. **Set goals**. Set professional and personal goals for yourself that are realistic and attainable.

13. **Take breaks**. Overdoing it can make you feel physically and mentally exhausted. Take breaks when you can and be easy on yourself.

14. **Continue your research**. Knowing the latest research and findings on chronic kidney disease can offer hope for the future and show you that others are working on finding new treatment options for people with your condition.

15. **Find healthy stress management techniques.** Learn healthy ways to manage your stress, anxiety,

and depression. Address any issues before they become too overwhelming to manage.

Your 1st Year Plan-Simple Tips to Lower Stress

The first year is always the hardest when it comes to dealing with the stress and anxiety that can come from being diagnosed, and living with, chronic kidney disease. In the first year you're still trying to process the news, as well as learning to adjust to your new normal.

It's no wonder that you are feeling a little out of sorts.

Over time, negativity and stress can drain you of the emotional energy necessary for you to live a fulfilling life. When you experience worsening symptoms, it can trigger negative thoughts that can make things worse.

The Role Of Stress And Anxiety

Unfortunately, stress and anxiety can have very real physical, as well as emotional, effects on the body. Learning to control your stress levels in the first year of your diagnosis will help set the stage for how you manage your stress and anxiety for years to come. Learning healthy stress relieving techniques is crucial.

Stress is basically the body's reaction to any change that requires a physical or emotional adjustment. Being diagnosed and learning to live with chronic kidney disease is certainly an adjustment that can cause stress. Although some stress is good, since it can keep you motivated and alert, too much can make you physically ill.

A negative stress reaction can lead to all kinds of physical ailments. Distress, which is what happens when stress continues without any relief, can cause:

- Sexual dysfunction
- Elevated blood pressure
- Chest pain
- Headaches
- Insomnia
- Digestive trouble

Emotional problems that can result from too much stress include anxiety, depression, and panic attacks. Elevated stress levels can aggravate symptoms of chronic kidney disease and has been linked to other medical conditions such as heart disease and even some forms of cancer.

It's important to address high levels of stress as quickly as possible. It has been shown that those with various types of chronic illnesses experience the highest risk of depressive symptoms within the first two years. Certain physical limitations imposed by chronic illnesses can lead to depression and depression can make your overall physical condition worse.

Tips To Lower Your Stress Levels

Learning to lower your stress levels in a healthy way is important. Part of controlling your stress means gaining a sense of control over your life and body.

1. **Educate yourself.** Gain the information you need in order to be informed about your healthcare.

2. **Make environmental changes**. Organize your home and work space so that daily living tasks are easier to manage.

3. **Find support**. Support groups, online or in the local area, can be utilized as a means of finding others who are experiencing similar symptoms and lifestyle changes. Online support groups for chronic illnesses, include chronic kidney disease, can be found on many websites including:

   Daily Strength Online Support: www.dailystrength.org

   The American Association of Kidney Patients: www.aakp.org

   The National Kidney Foundation: http://www.kidney.org/

   MedHelp Online Health Community: http://www.medhelp.org/

4. **Follow through with treatment.** Make the necessary lifestyle changes that you need in order to be as healthy as possible. Take all medications and follow through with all treatment plans including dietary changes.

5. **Learn your symptoms**. Learn any triggers that can make your condition worse. For instance, some situations might be extremely stressful and cause your blood pressure to increase. Avoid these when possible.

6. **Communicate with others**. ommunicate with your loved ones or your doctors about how you feel. Bring up any changes you might be experiencing, no matter how small and insignificant you think they are.

7. **Learn new stress management techniques**. Practice meditating, creative visualizing, or deep breathing exercises to help you manage your stress and anxiety. You can also use hobbies as a way to cope with stress and to relax your mind. Painting or woodworking, for instance, can offer you a task that can be relaxing and enjoyable.

8. **Change your outlook**. Try to change your negative thought patterns by changing your perspective to make it a more positive one. Look at what you can do instead of what you cannot do.

9. **Find new interests**. Continue to challenge yourself so that you are finding new interests and setting goals, no matter how small, for yourself. Have dreams and strive for them.

10. **Face your emotions**. Instead of shying away from and/or ignoring your emotions, learn to identify and resolve them when you can. When you're feeling angry, try to understand why

you're feeling that way. It might be something that is fixable. If it's not fixable, then give yourself permission to feel what you are feeling, unjustifiable or not, to alleviate your stress.

A New Approach To Your Health

It's now important to focus on your health. Understand that your emotional health can affect your physical health. How you feel emotionally can have a very strong effect on how you feel physically. A positive approach can manifest in a healthier wellbeing.

If you're in the advanced stages of chronic kidney disease or submitting to regular dialysis then you might feel as though you have lost some of your prior independence. These feelings can take a toll on your self-esteem, self-worth, and self-confidence. Feeling dependent on others can cause you to feel a loss of power and control that you once had. You might even impose blame on yourself for having chronic kidney disease in the first place.

Taking a new approach to your health is imperative. You can't just focus on the physical symptoms, you have to look at your emotional wellbeing. Think of your body as a complete entity that needs to be fed and nurtured, both physically and mentally.

In order to take care of yourself and your medical condition you have to learn to let go and find acceptance in your life. Once you're able to relinquish the old definition of yourself and life prior to diagnosis, you can redefine who you are and create new meaning for yourself and purpose beyond your chronic kidney disease.

Working with Your Doctors

Building a good relationship with your healthcare team is important since it will affect how you relate to them in terms of your treatment and ongoing care. It's important to find a doctor you trust and with whom you feel comfortable. Not only does your doctor see to your needs; he/she must also have a good rapport with you so that you feel comfortable going to him/her with questions and concerns.

What You Might Expect

What treatment options and doctors you might see depends on the level or degree of your kidney disease. Those in the early stages (Stages 1 and 2) do not need to see their doctors as often as those who are in advanced kidney disease stages.

Someone with Stage 2 chronic kidney disease has mild kidney damage and is probably without symptoms. You may have found out you have kidney disease while you were being tested for something else. Simple lifestyle changes to regulate blood sugar and blood pressure levels may be enough to keep the disease from progressing rapidly. You might still have regular testing for protein in the urine and serum creatinine which can show if the kidney damage is progressing. A renal diet is an excellent way to slow the progression of your chronic kidney failure. Some people facing chronic kidney disease see dietitians in order to help them create healthy diets so that they can practice self-care at home. Other patients may visit counselors or psychiatrists if they need help with emotional or mental issues.

In most cases, you'll work with more than one doctor when it comes to managing your chronic kidney disease. Some of the healthcare professionals who are able to diagnose and treat chronic kidney disease include:

- Family medicine physicians
- Internists
- Nephrologists
- Pediatricians
- Nurse practitioners
- Physician assistants (PA)

How often you visit your doctor, or doctors, will depend upon how far your kidney disease has progressed. Patients in Stage 3 normally visit their doctor every 3-6 months. At this time, blood tests for creatinine, hemoglobin, calcium, sodium, potassium, and phosphorus levels are carried out to see how well your kidneys are functioning. You may start limiting the protein in your diet. Doctors will also monitor other conditions you might have which can affect kidney function such as high blood pressure, heart disease, and diabetes.

More than likely, you will be sent to a nephrologist for treatment once you have been diagnosed with chronic kidney disease and are in Stage 3. A nephrologist is a kidney specialist. A nephrologist can examine you and perform lab tests to gather information about your condition to offer the best advice for treatment. The primary goal is to help you keep your kidneys working as long and as well as possible.

Those in Stage 4 normally visit their doctor at least every three months. You're monitored at this time and the nephrologist will also help prepare you for dialysis or a kidney transplant. In Stage 4, you prepare for a few different treatment options that are available as you approach End Stage Renal Disease (ESRD). These can include hemodialysis, peritoneal dialysis (PD) or a kidney transplant. If you are in need of a dialysis access site or if you are having a kidney transplant, you might be referred to a surgeon.

In Stage 5 kidney disease, a person has end stage renal disease. At this point, the kidneys have lost nearly all their ability to do their job effectively. Dialysis or a transplant is necessary. You may get on the transplant list at this time, and you will be working closely with your health care team to start dialysis and improve your health. At this point, many people feel exhausted, and starting dialysis actually makes them feel much better after the initial change.

Being Your Own Advocate

No matter how good your healthcare provider or team is and how comfortable you are with them, you are always going to have to be your own advocate! Take an active role in your health care. This means that you'll need to learn the medical terminology that is used for the various aspects of chronic kidney disease, you'll have to voice your concerns when it feels like you're not being heard, and you'll need to ask questions to ensure that you understand what's going on.

Some of the questions that you might ask your doctor include:

- What is causing my kidney disease?

- How will kidney disease affect me?

- What is my prognosis?

- Which treatment option is best for me at this time and why?

- Are there any medications that I should or should not take?

- Is there a special diet I need to follow?

- Is there an exercise plan that is right for me?

- Would it help if I lost weight or quit smoking?

- Is there a chance I will need dialysis? Will it be painful?

- What will happen if I don't get dialysis?

- Am I going to need a kidney transplant?

Be an active participant in all of your appointments. Listen to what your doctor says and if you don't understand a diagnosis or treatment then be sure to ask him/her questions. Doctors see a lot of patients during the day so it's up to you to be your own advocate. Bring up any issues you've been having and make sure you leave feeling satisfied with your visit.

If you have trouble remembering what you want to talk about, make a list and take that with you. Take your partner, a family member, or a positive friend with you to your appointments, too. Four ears are better than two. Take a notepad with your questions for your doctors that you have been writing down and write out important notes and instructions.

Being Sick in a Healthy World

It is not easy being sick in a world that appears to be healthy. There are new challenges to be faced every day, whether it's sticking to a new diet or trying to maneuver through a shopping center with less energy than you had before. It's also challenging to go through life with an invisible illness and symptoms that aren't always understood. It is possible to forge new, stronger bonds with the people you love, and to find new ways of enjoying life and coping with your setbacks.

The People Around You

Kidney disease comes with different symptoms and treatment options and you can have other related medical conditions. These can have their own symptoms and management challenges. You might find that your family and friends are profoundly affected by what you are going through. As a result, they may end up needing their own support. Although you are technically the one going through the physical changes, your loved ones can also go through emotional turmoil as they attempt to adjust to the changes that have occurred as they watch someone they love become ill.

And for some others there are significant role changes and changes in responsibilities. This can overwhelm the caregiver, and cause feelings of helplessness to you.

As your kidney disease progresses there can be fear and sadness as the image of yourself may change. You might also suffer from emotional, physical and financial drains. Your loved ones or caregivers may feel lonely and isolated.

As a result, it's important for primary caregivers to receive support and guidance when necessary.

Dealing with the emotions of others can seem like an extra burden to you and you might feel guilty or even angry. Effective communication is important and sometimes those with chronic kidney disease find that seeking outside counsel is helpful as they and their loved ones learn to deal with new setbacks and stressors.

Managing Your Care

If you are still in the early stages of kidney disease, managing your care and working with your doctors is essential to giving you a better quality of life and ensuring that your kidneys continue to function well. A lot of the damage caused by CKD occurs early, when interventions may be very effective. You might find that you now have new limitations and guidelines to follow, especially if you are in advanced stages of kidney disease.

So what does this mean in terms of diet, exercise, and medications?

Using preventive measures to ensure that you don't face any unnecessary illnesses which might intensify your situation is important. This might mean getting vaccinations against the flu and pneumonia. You'll also need to monitor any other health issues you have which could include monitoring your blood pressure, sugar levels, and protein in your urine.

Certain medications may need to be stopped and avoided. Diuretics, NSAIDS, and drugs that are capable of causing interstitial nephritis, like penicillin, will be reviewed by your doctor to see if you should avoid them or use them with caution.

A renal diet is needed once you enter stage 3, and this might mean eliminating or adding different foods. Foods that have little sodium are best and foods that are healthy for your heart such as fruits, vegetables, and certain types of fish. You might need to eat less protein since it can cause your kidneys to work harder.

If you must limit your potassium intake then you'll need to drink apple juice or cranberry juice rather than orange juice. You might need to limit phosphorus which means that you should choose light-colored soda such as lemon-lime, iced tea and lemonade. All of this information should be considered to be general and it is recommended that you consult with your doctor or nephrologist before changing your diet. If you are interested in learning more about a renal diet, please check out our website at www.renaldiethq.com

Self-Care

Developing a sense of self-care is important when you're living with chronic kidney disease. It can mean different things but usually involves being aware of your own health needs and knowing what actions you must take to stay as healthy as possible. It can mean being your own advocate, developing healthy habits, attending all of your medical appointments, making healthy lifestyle choices, and knowing if and when you should seek treatment.

Although you might need to rely on medication for some problem areas, there is some self-care that you can perform at home on your own which can greatly affect your quality of life and keep your condition from progressing at a faster rate. Your doctor should speak to you about treating the problems that might have damaged your kidneys.

Many people with chronic kidney disease, have high blood pressure, heart disease or diabetes. If you have high blood pressure or heart disease, then you might need to take medications to help lower it. These can work to lower your blood pressure and may help keep your kidney disease from progressing. However, regular physical activity and a healthy renal diet can work to lower your blood pressure as well. Engaging in a healthy exercise plan can help your emotional health, too, since your body produces endorphins when you exercise and these are nature's "happy" hormones.

If you also have diabetes then you will work with your doctor to find ways to keep your blood sugar levels regulated. This might mean taking more medication. It could also mean getting more exercise and eliminating certain foods from your diet. Many diabetics must perform blood sugar tests on themselves throughout the day. By learning to do this you can keep an eye on your sugar levels and will be able to alert someone if they are elevated. Eating a renal diet and making a meal plan is another of the things that can help keep your condition from progressing at a faster rate.

Since smoking can damage the kidneys, it is important that you quit smoking. Not only is it harmful to your kidneys, but it can elevate your blood pressure and even interfere with certain medications. It also affects your heart and is considered a cause of heart disease.

Living With An Invisible Illness

Most people are not able to tell that you have chronic kidney disease simply by looking at you. Since the early stages might not have any symptoms at all, and the later stages have symptoms that could be signs of something else, chronic kidney disease can be classified as an "invisible" illness.

Living with an invisible illness presents its own unique challenges. You might already feel as though you are alone in a world full of healthy people. Even if you are not bound to your house and are still able to work, you might feel lonely and isolated. Talking to friends or co-workers about your medical condition can be uncomfortable and you might feel hesitant to do so.

Many people with invisible chronic illnesses are afraid of sounding like they are complaining too much so they minimize their symptoms. This can lead to a break in communication and more feelings of isolation. Fatigue can be one of the major symptoms of chronic kidney disease. It's not uncommon to find that your circle of close friends grows smaller over time. Some people drift away, unable to keep up a friendship with someone who isn't as available to socialize like they did in the past.

On the positive side, however, you might also find that you're able to forge stronger bonds with those you weren't as close to in the past and you might meet new people who can act as a support system. Some people find that their communication becomes stronger and clearer since they must articulate their needs and symptoms more effectively with their healthcare provider and this transcends into their personal life as well.

Coping With Ongoing Issues

Although the symptoms of early stages of kidney disease can be quiet, in later stages some of the symptoms can be tough to deal with. Sometimes you must treat the symptoms individually and this can present its own difficulties.

Fatigue is one of the most common symptoms of chronic kidney disease. It is sometimes caused by anemia so talking to your healthcare provider about iron supplements might help alleviate some of the tiredness and lack of energy. Fatigue can cause problems because you might over-exert yourself quickly and find that you don't always have the energy to perform activities that you once enjoyed. Learning to take breaks and to go easy on yourself is important.

Fluid buildup is another common symptom in kidney disease. Over time the kidneys can lose their ability to control the amount of fluid in your body. This can cause swelling in the hands, face, feet, and legs. You should also talk to your doctor about ways to relive fluid buildup and swelling. When your legs or feet are swollen it can make walking and moving around painful and difficult. Sometimes it's even necessary to use a cane, walker, or a wheelchair.

Many people find that they have symptoms that are more obviously connected to their kidneys and these symptoms can be embarrassing and problematic. Frequent urination, for instance, is a symptom that is common with kidney disease. It might mean that you have to get up several times in the night to use the restroom or that you have to make frequent trips when you're out in public. Some people are afraid to go out in public for long because they might have an accident.

Insomnia is another common problem associated with kidney disease. Trouble sleeping is a particularly aggravating issue because adequate sleep is necessary for overall positive wellbeing. If you don't get enough sleep your body has trouble fighting off infections and you can feel even more rundown and fatigued. Lack of proper sleep can also lead to depression or worsen the symptoms of existing depression.

Coping with some of the ongoing medical issues associated with kidney disease can be hard. This is one reason you must establish good rapport with your healthcare providers. If you're experiencing any problems that are affecting your quality of life then speak to them about what might be done about it. In some cases, making simple dietary changes or taking certain medication and/or supplements might help remedy the problems that you're facing. Remember, NEVER stop or change medication without discussing it with your healthcare professionals.

Love Yourself and Conquer Life

People who must live with a chronic illness have good days and bad days. There are ups and downs and highs and lows. Addressing all the feelings that come with living with a chronic condition and giving yourself permission to feel them is a step in learning to conquer your disease and love the new you.

It's easy to feel guilty when you're living with something like chronic kidney disease. You might feel guilty that your lifestyle could have attributed to your illness and you could also feel guilty at the idea of placing burden on your loved ones. Some people even feel guilty at the idea of feeling bad. After all, you *want* to be positive. Anger and helplessness might be emotions that are hard to deal with and, therefore, the presence of these emotions could make you feel like you're doing something wrong.

Just remember that you are human.

Loving Yourself In Spite Of Your Illness

One of the toughest parts of learning to live with chronic kidney disease is learning to love your body. It's not easy. After all, you may feel that your body has betrayed you. You took care of it to the best of your ability.

Learning to love yourself while living with a chronic illness isn't easy. It requires effort, concentration, and belief in yourself. Although you'll get lots of advice from family, friends, and doctors; it's up to you to know what you need.

Having chronic kidney disease allows you to get to know your body and mind like never before. It also offers you the chance for reflection and self realization. Caring for your soul and mind is just as important as caring for your body.

Learning that your self-worth and value do not consist of what you are physically able to do, but who you are as a person is essential on this journey.

Your illness is not you. It's a part of who you are, but it isn't all of who you are.

Take things a little at a time. You'll eventually learn to accept your situation as it is. That situation may change over time, especially if you progress into later stages of kidney disease and diet and medication are no longer enough to manage it. Taking things one day at a time and as they come can help you avoid feeling overwhelmed and anxious. Remember you might step back through the stages of grief as your condition changes.

Learn to take pride in your accomplishments, no matter how small and insignificant they might feel at the time. Some days, you'll accomplish a lot. Other days, simply getting out of bed and getting dressed might be an accomplishment. Develop a new yardstick in which to measure your success. In the past, you might have been able to go the entire day without a nap. With fatigue being present, this might not be possible. Instead of accepting your new limitation as a failure, make your goal a little smaller and more realistic. Rather than be upset that you have to lay down and rest, consider that as a way to pamper yourself and be in a good mood for later in the day. And then feel good about yourself when you do it – Lots of people take an afternoon siesta!

Above all, learn to have compassion for yourself. You will find that the love you develop for your new normal will extend into other areas of your life, and even affect your personal relationships in a positive way.

Some people find that in the wake of a chronic illness, they actually develop a greater appreciation for themselves, their lives, and the people around them. Joy and possibility still remains in life, as long as you remain open to them.

Conclusion

Although being diagnosed with chronic kidney disease might momentarily take the wind out of your sails, it doesn't mean an end to the quality of life you wish to have. In fact, you actually have the chance to achieve significant insight into yourself as you move through and cope with the different facets of the disease.

Of course, having a chronic condition of any kind means that you will face challenges along the way. From time to time you may have setbacks. There will be some times that you are able to cope more effectively with your condition than others. There might be days when you want to throw in the towel.

It's important not to give up while you're on your journey. Learn new ways of gaining compassion and respect for yourself and your "new normal" as you redefine and restructure your life around your illness.

You'll also learn new standards in which to measure your accomplishments and expectations. Although you might face limitations that you didn't have to work around in the past, part of rising above your condition means that you recognize that you are more than simply your body and its symptoms. You are able to realize that life can have purpose and meaning even though your body might impose limitations upon your actions.

Instead of seeing yourself without your chronic kidney disease, try to accept yourself disease for what you are and live in the moment. Take control over what you can; your attitude and outlook on life.

Like grief, adapting to your chronic illness is a process with stages that aren't always linear. You might arrive at acceptance, only to have a setback and experience depression. You'll continuously be challenged to revisit different emotions and issues. Learning healthy coping strategies can permit you to return to the place where you're dedicated to having the best quality of life.

In the face of adversity, it takes a lot of determination and strength to continue fighting. Congratulate and acknowledge yourself for possessing these qualities. Be gentle with yourself. Forgive yourself when you hit a rough patch. Healthy living has as much to do with the way that you think as it does the physical aspects of your health. When you are able to live your life in a meaningful way, you are creating a personal sense of self-worth. You *are* more than just your illness.

Next Steps

1. Think about the stages of grief and where you are in your understanding and feelings about your chronic kidney disease. Are you depressed or sad? Do you feel you have accepted the disease and you are ready to live with where you are now?

2. Have you spoken to members of your family about how they can help you? When you found out did you discuss what it means as a caregiver and talk about how your roles will change? It's time to do that now if you have not done it before. This is a fundamental shift in your relationship, and requires some discussion so that you both are on the same page.

3. Emotionally, you might be a wreck or you might be just fine. Identify where you are and how you are handling the stress. If you think you are handling it well, talk to your caregiver about his/her opinion. If you have taken some of your anger out on a caregiver with words or behavior, it's time to talk about it. Keeping it out in the open is key to working through the difficult times.

Other Titles By Mathea Ford:

Mathea Ford, Author Page (all books):

http://www.amazon.com/Mathea-Ford/e/B008E1E7IS/

The Kidney Friendly Diet Cookbook

http://www.amazon.com/Kidney-Friendly-Diet-Cookbook-PreDialysis-ebook/dp/B00BC7BGPI/

Create Your Own Kidney Diet Plan

http://www.amazon.com/Create-Your-Kidney-Diet-Plan-ebook/dp/B009PSN3R0/

Living with Chronic Kidney Disease - Pre-Dialysis

http://www.amazon.com/Living-Chronic-Kidney-Disease-Pre-Dialysis-ebook/dp/B008D8RSAQ/

Eating a Pre-Dialysis Kidney Diet - Calories, Carbohydrates, Fat & Protein, Secrets To Avoid Dialysis

http://www.amazon.com/Eating-Pre-Dialysis-Kidney-Diet-Carbohydrates-ebook/dp/B00DU2JCHM/

Eating a Pre-Dialysis Kidney Diet - Sodium, Potassium, Phosphorus and Fluids, A Kidney Disease Soluion

http://www.amazon.com/Eating-Pre-Dialysis-Kidney-Diet-Phosphorus-ebook/dp/B00E2U8VMS/

Eating Out On a Kidney Diet: Pre-dialysis and Diabetes: Ways To Enjoy Your Favorite Foods

http://www.amazon.com/Eating-Out-Kidney-Diet-Pre-dialysis/dp/0615928781/

Kidney Disease: Common Labs and Medical Terminology: The Patient's Perspective

http://www.amazon.com/Kidney-Disease-Terminology-Perspective-Pre-Dialysis/dp/0615931804/

Dialysis: Treatment Options for the Progression to End Stage Renal Disease

http://www.amazon.com/Dialysis-Treatment-Options-Progression-Disease/dp/0615932258/

Mindful Eating For A Pre-Dialysis Kidney Diet: Healthy Attitudes Toward Food and Life

http://www.amazon.com/Mindful-Eating-Pre-Dialysis-Kidney-Diet/dp/0615933475/

CPSIA information can be obtained
at www.ICGtesting.com
Printed in the USA
LVOW13s1128180917
549111LV00006B/1285/P